Copyright © Stephanie Baker

All rights reserved. No part of this book may be reproduced, scanned or distributed in any printed or electronic form without permission. Please do not participate in or encourage piracy of copyrighted materials in violation of the author's rights. Purchase only authorized editions.

1
EGG LASAGNE LOW CARB

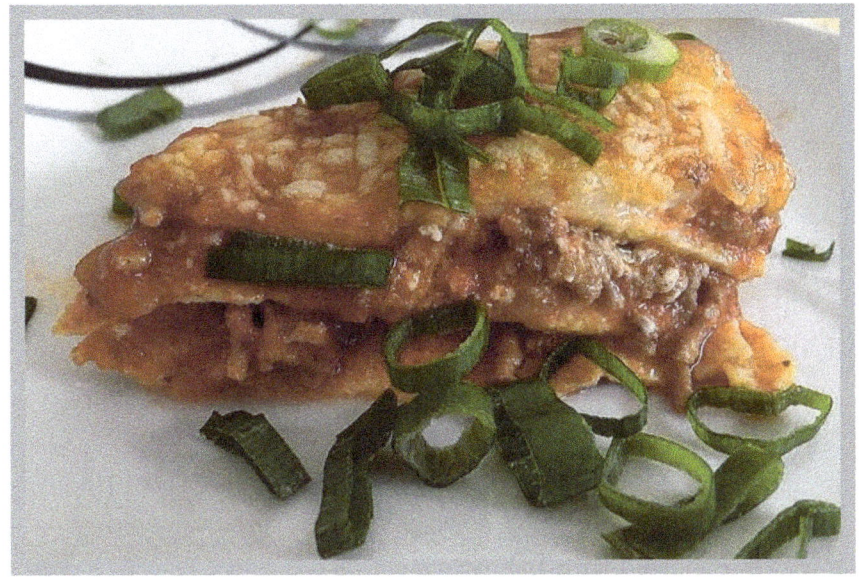

45 MIN.
Simple

. . .

INGREDIENTS

6 Servings

- 1 cupcreme fraiche cheese
- 500 gminced meat
- onion (noun)
- 1 cantomatoes, chunky, 400 g, or fresh
- 1 pck.Tomatoes, strained, 500 g
- 200 gcheese, grated
- 100 mlcream
- 1 pinchflour
- Somethingoil
- N. B.Herbs, e.g. B. Oregano, basil, thyme
- Salt and pepper
- 6thegg (s)
- Somethingnutmeg

PREPARATION

1. Approximate working time: 45 minutes
2. Approximate cooking / baking time: 20 minutes
3. 1 hour and 5 minutes is the approximate total time.
4. Break open the six eggs and whisk them together for the lasagne dishes. Place the egg mixture on a baking sheet lined with baking paper and spread it out as evenly as possible. Place the tray in a hot oven and cook the eggs for 80 to 100 minutes on top/bottom heat. Take a look now and then, and be happy to

scatter the mixture equally over the entire sheet in between, resulting in an even tray.

5. Peel and chop the onions for the minced meat filling, then fry them until translucent. Add the beef that has been minced. Season the meat with salt and pepper before frying it. Then add the sliced or fresh tomatoes, as well as the strained tomatoes, to deglaze. Season with salt and pepper to taste, then set aside to steep. I like to use oregano, basil, and thyme, in fact, anything green and readily available.

6. Heat a little oil and stir in the flour with the tip of a knife to make the bechamel sauce. Deglaze with the cream and a splash of water, if necessary, and mix until smooth. Salt, pepper, and nutmeg to taste. Place the crème fraîche in a separate bowl and set it aside.

7. Break the egg mixture into slices that fit the size of the baking dish. In the baking dish, separate layers of minced meat sauce, béchamel sauce, and lasagne dishes. The bechamel should be the last sheet, followed by a crispy topping.

8. Then bake all until the cheese is golden brown in a hot oven set to 180° c top/bottom pressure. Since all of the ingredients are prepared ahead of time, the baking time can be changed, and i prefer it after about 20 minutes.

② ZUCCHINI PASTA LOW CARB

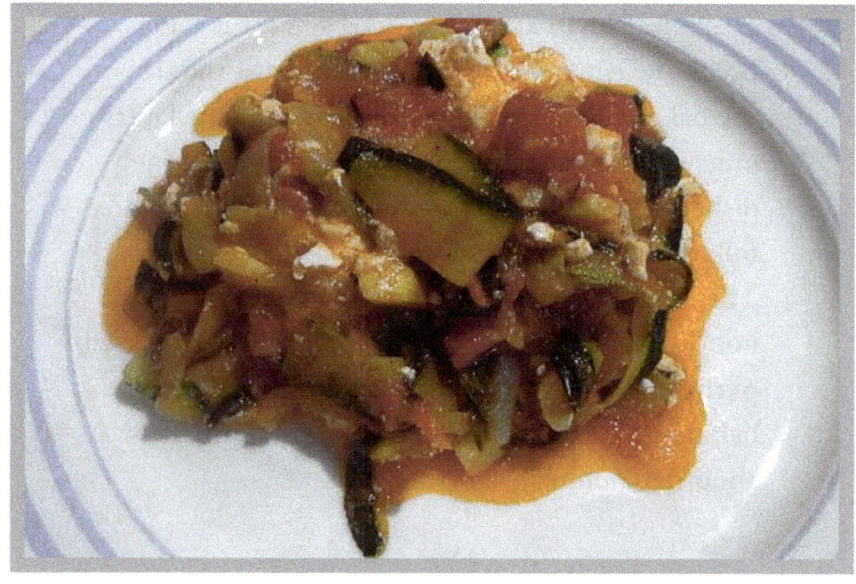

25 MIN.
Simple
449 kcal

KETO PASTA

. . .

INGREDIENTS

2 Servings

- 4 m.-largezucchini
- 1 cantomato (s), chopped
- onion (noun)
- 1 packagefeta cheese
- Somethingsalt and pepper
- 1 toe / ngarlic, or garlic powder
- Somethingoil or other fat

NUTRITIONAL VALUES per serving

Kcal

449

Protein

25.07 g

Fat

30.57 g

Carbohydrate

16.29 g

PREPARATION

1. Approximate working time: 25 minutes
2. Time to cook / bake: approx. 1 hour 15 minutes
3. Approximate total time: Time: 40 minutes

4. Remove the ends of the zucchini and wash it. Peel the zucchini lengthwise into strips with a vegetable peeler or potato peeling knife. The "ribbon noodles" are made in this manner. Peel all the way down to the heart. The remainder can be discarded or cut into small pieces and added to the sauce. Sprinkle salt over the ribbon noodles in a sieve. The water in the zucchini is removed in this way. Break the onion into small pieces after peeling it. Pat the "ribbon noodles" dry with a kitchen towel after a while.
5. In a pan, heat some oil and cook the zucchini strips with the onions. Toss in the tomatoes and feta cheese, sliced. Combine the pressed garlic (or garlic powder) and the remaining spices in a mixing bowl. Enable the mixture to boil for a few minutes, or the zucchini may become too soft.

③
LOW-CARB NOODLES MADE FROM CHICKPEA FLOUR, WITHOUT EGG

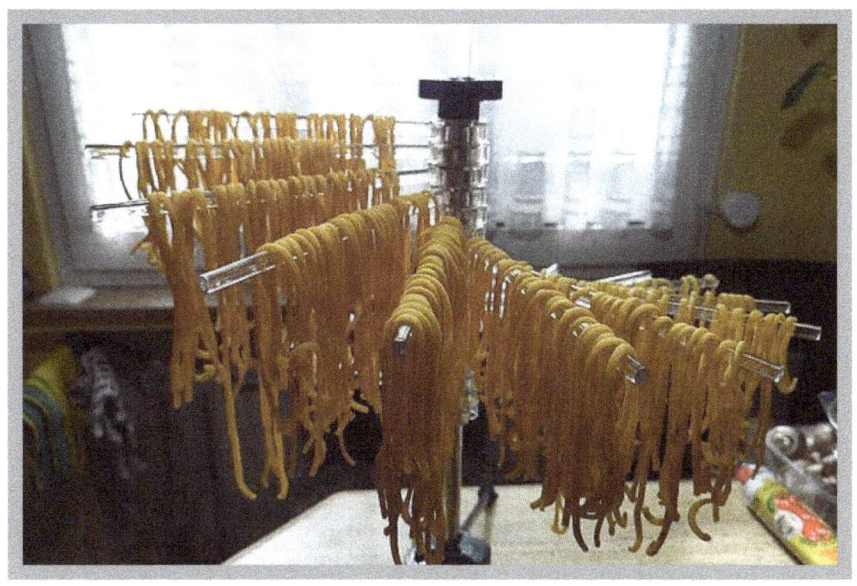

20 MIN.

Normal

. . .

INGREDIENTS

4 Servings

- 380 g chickpea flour
- 20 g gluten
- 15 g xanthan gum
- 150 ml water, ice cold
- 1 ½ tsp, heaped salt

PREPARATION

1. Approximate working time: 20 minutes
2. Approximate rest time: 2 hours
3. Complete time: 2 hours and 20 minutes
4. Dissolve the salt absolutely in the water and uniformly combine the dry ingredients.
5. Start the pasta maker by pouring the flour mixture into it. Slowly pour in the salt water (over 2 minutes). Just use enough water to keep the dough loose and grainy. 145 mL is usually sufficient, but the exact amount varies slightly depending on the flour and environmental conditions.
6. Allow at least two hours for the pasta to dry before cooking. Noodles that have been fully dried can also be stored without issue.

4

MEDITERRANEAN LOW-CARB NOODLES WITH BELL PEPPER, ROCKET AND MINCED MEAT

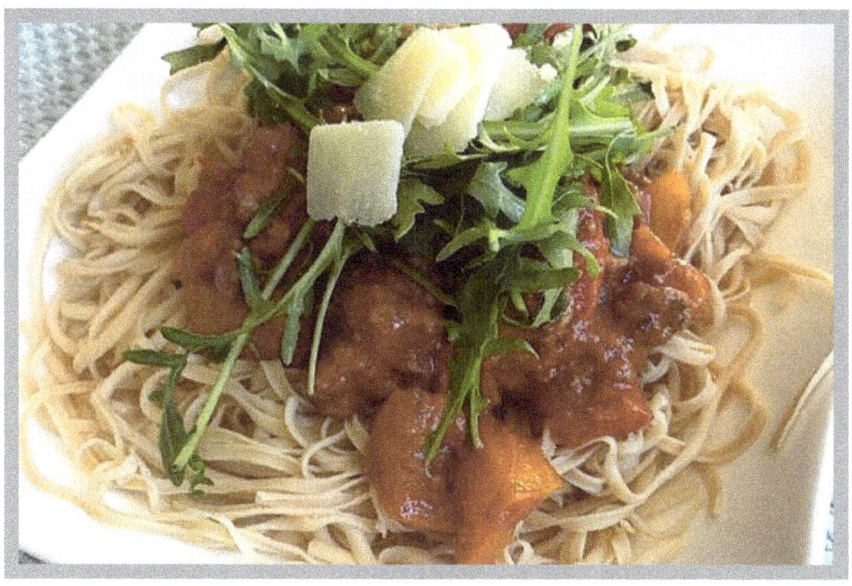

30 MIN.

Normal

415 kcal

. . .

INGREDIENTS

3 Servings

- 200 gspaghetti (soybean spaghetti)
- 350 gtartare or minced meat
- 1 pck. Tomatoes, happened
- 2bell pepper
- 2shallot (noun)
- garlic cloves)
- Salt and pepper
- Arugula
- Parmesan
- Olive oil

PREPARATION

1. Approximate working time: 30 minutes
2. Approximate cooking / baking time: 20 minutes
3. Approximate total time: 50 minutes
4. The peppers should be cored, chopped, and lightly browned in olive oil. Remove the fried pepper pieces and set them aside.
5. In the same pan, brown the minced meat. Chop the peeled shallots and garlic cloves, then add them to the pan and cook until they're translucent. Return the pepper parts to the pot and deglaze with the

tomatoes. Bring to a boil and season to taste with salt and pepper.
6. In the meantime, add salted water to the pot and, as soon as it boils, cook the soy noodles according to package directions, then drain.
7. Assemble the pasta and sauce on the plate, then top with a tiny handful of rocket and a sprinkling of parmesan.
8. Hint: Regular spaghetti can be used instead of low-carb noodles. The minced meat is actually omitted by vegetarians.

5
LOW CARBOHYDRATE KOHLRABI LASAGNA

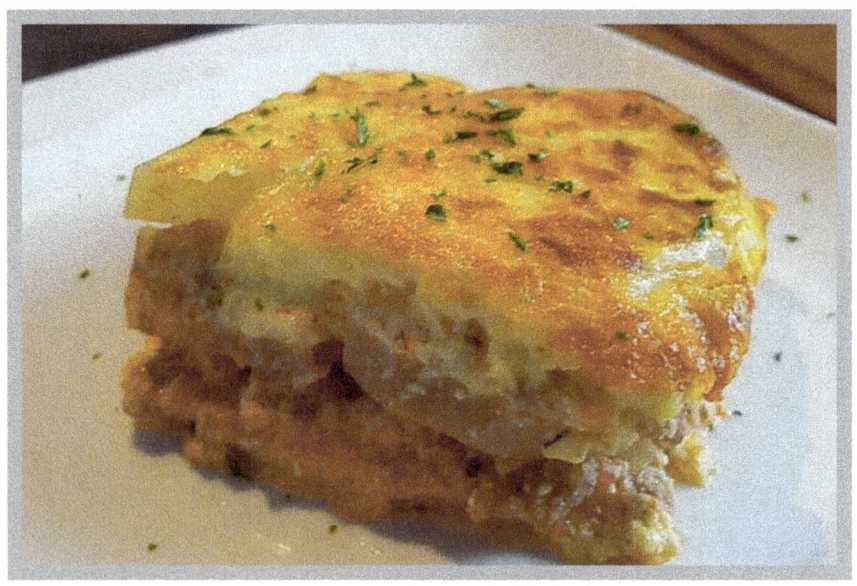

30 MINUTES.
Easy

. . .

INGREDIENTS

4th Servings

- Kohlrabi 1 m high
- Saltwater
- 500 g minced meat
- 500 g tomatoes, it happened
- 3 carrots
- 1 small onion
- 3 heaped teaspoons of ajvar, smooth
- mushrooms
- 200 g of grated cheese
- 1 cup of fresh cream cheese
- salt and pepper
- Cayenne pepper
- Paprika powder, nobly sweet
- Topping for pizza or topping for pasta

PREPARATION

1. Working time approx. 30 minutes
2. Cooking time / cooking time approx. 30 minutes
3. Total time approx. 1 hour
4. Peel the kohlrabi, cut into thin slices and cook in salted boiling water for 10 minutes. Cut the remaining vegetables into small pieces.
5. Preheat the oven to 180 ° C (convection). In the meantime, fry the ground beef and season with salt, pepper, cayenne pepper and paprika powder.
6. Add the chopped vegetables, tomatoes, and ajvar.

7. Season the sauce with pizza or pasta toppings and other toppings. Let simmer briefly.
8. Then, as usual, place a layer of lasagne in a baking dish. Start with the sauce, then sprinkle the kohlrabi slices, using the sauce and fresh cream as the final layer, and sprinkle the cheese on top.
9. About. Place in the oven for 10-15 minutes until the cheese has the desired degree of browning.

6

LOW CARB ZUCCHINI CARROT NOODLES WITH PRAWNS

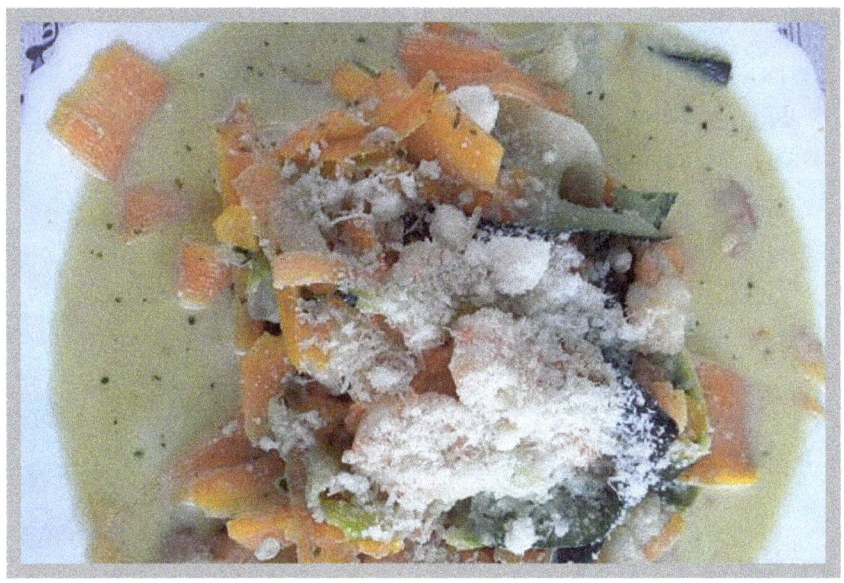

10 MINS.

Normal

528 kcal

. . .

INGREDIENTS

4th Servings

- 1 m. Large zucchini
- carrots
- 500 g prawns)
- 400 ml whipped cream
- 3 tsp, knit. Herbs, Italian
- salt and pepper
- Butter or oil

Nutritional values per serving

Kcal

528

protein

27.99 g

fat

39.02 g

carbohydrate

17.07 g

PREPARATION

1. Working time approx. 10 minutes
2. Cooking time / cooking time approx. 25 minutes
3. Total time approx. 35 minutes

4. Wash the carrots and zucchini. Peel the carrots, then peel the strips with the peeler. Do the same with the unpeeled zucchini. Blanch the carrot and zucchini strips in salted water for about 30 minutes. 3 minutes.
5. In a pan or saucepan, melt butter or oil. Fry the prawns for a couple of minutes, then add the carrot and zucchini strips and cook for another 5 minutes, stirring occasionally. Then add the cream and season with salt and pepper. As a last step, add the Italian herbs and simmer for about 10-15 minutes.
6. Sprinkle with parmesan or basil to serve.

⬤7
LOW CARB NOODLES WITH SKYR

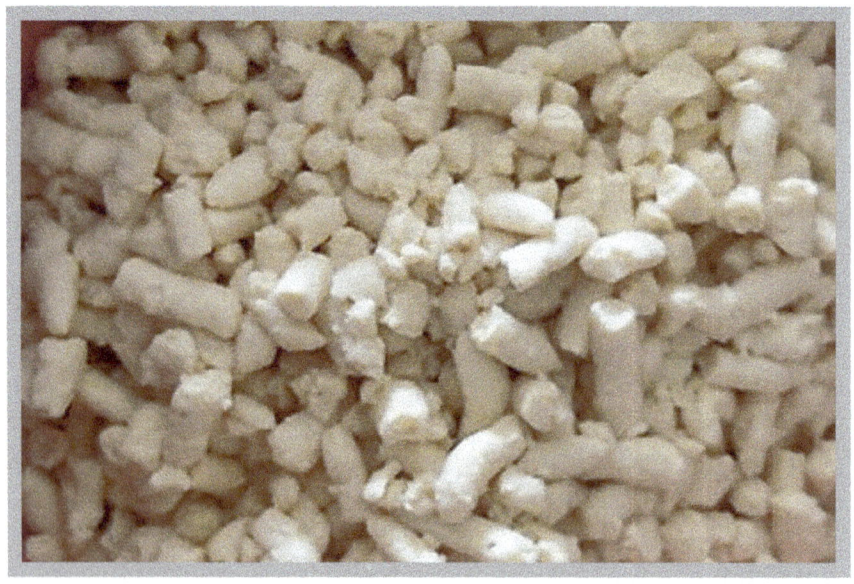

10 MINUTES.
Easy

. . .

INGREDIENTS

2 servings

- 250 grams of skyr
- 2 eggs)
- 4 tablespoons of guar gum

PREPARATION

1. Processing time about 10 minutes.
2. Rest time about 10 minutes.
3. Cooking time/cooking approx. 10 minutes
4. Total time about 30 minutes
5. Beat the eggs and skyr first. Then work the sifted guar gum, stirring constantly.
6. The dough must rest for 10 minutes before rolling it out and cutting it into thin dough strips.
7. Put the prepared pasta in boiling water for about 10 minutes. Drain and postpone.

8

SPICY CARROT NOODLES WITH PARMESAN - LOW CARB

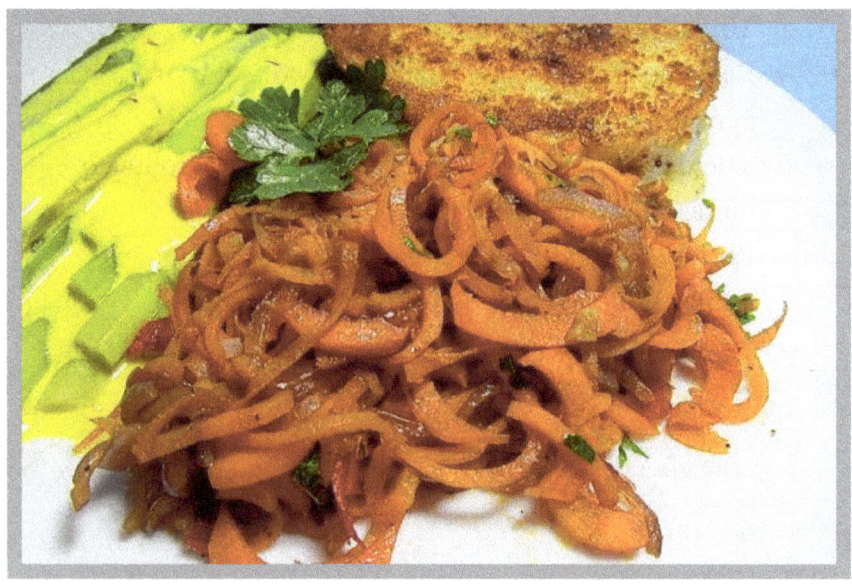

15 MINUTES.
normal
400 kcal

INGREDIENTS

1 serving

- large carrots
- ½ small chili, alternatively chili powder as needed
- 1 onion
- 1 clove of garlic)
- 30 g of grated Parmesan cheese
- 1 tablespoon of balsamic vinegar
- 1 tablespoon of olive oil
- N. B. Chopped parsley
- salt and pepper

Nutritional values per serving
Kcal
400
protein
15.29 g
Fat
17.42 g
carbohydrate
44.54 g

PREPARATION

1. Processing time about 15 minutes

2. Cooking time / cooking approx. 15 minutes
3. Total time aboutAbout 30 minutes in total
4. A pot of salted water should be brought to a boil.

1. In the meantime, use the peeler to cut the carrots into "ribbon noodles". Pour boiling water into the pot and cook for about 3-4 minutes until al dente.
2. Peel the onions and cut them into rings, peel and dice the garlic clove. In a big skillet, heat 1 tablespoon olive oil and fry the onion rings and garlic until clear.
3. Drain the carrots while you collect the cooking water. Add the carrots to the onions with a little boiling water and sauté for a few minutes. Add some boiling water if necessary. After about 5 minutes, add the balsamic vinegar and season with salt and pepper. Sprinkle with Parmesan and serve sprinkled with a little parsley.

9
LOW-CARB LASAGNA OF KOHLRABI AND SPINACH

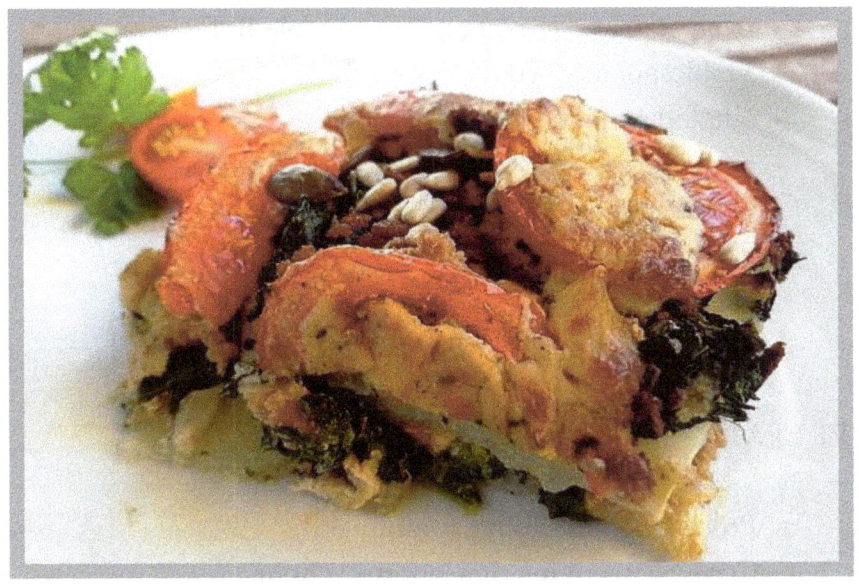

35 MIN.
Easy
430 kcal

. . .

INGREDIENTS

4 servings

- 750 g of spinach, frozen or fresh
- 1 kg of kohlrabi
- 4. tomatoes)
- 2 onions (noun)
- 2 cloves of garlic)
- 3 tablespoons of butter
- 3 tablespoons of flour
- 500 ml of milk
- 250 ml of water
- 150 g of grated cheese, p. For example B. Edam
- 2 tablespoons of sunflower seeds
- salt and pepper
- nutmeg
- Petroleum
- Fat for the shape

PREPARATION

1. Processing time about 35 minutes
2. Cooking / cooking time approx. 1 hour
3. Total time about 1 hour and 35 minutes
4. Divide the fresh spinach, wash it well and drain. Thaw frozen spinach and drain well.

5. Peel and wash the kohlrabi, cut into thin slices and cook in salted water for 2-3 minutes.
6. Meanwhile, toast the sunflower seeds in a fat-free skillet until golden brown.

1. Onions and garlic should be peeled and finely chopped. In a saucepan, heat a drizzle of oil and sauté half of the onions and garlic until clear. Cook the spinach until it starts to flake. Season with salt, pepper, and nutmeg to taste.
2. Heat the butter in a saucepan and sauté the rest of the onions and garlic. Add the flour and brown. Add the milk and water, bring to a boil and simmer for about 3 minutes. Season with salt, pepper and nutmeg.
3. Wash the tomatoes, remove the stalk and cut them into slices.
4. A 20 x 30 cm pan with sauce, kohlrabi, spinach, and tomatoes alternated. Finish with the tomatoes and sauce, then grate the cheese on top.
5. Pre-heat oven for 175 degrees Celsius and bake for 40 minutes.
6. Sprinkle with sunflower seeds and serve.

10
LOW CARB SPAGHETTI CARBONARA

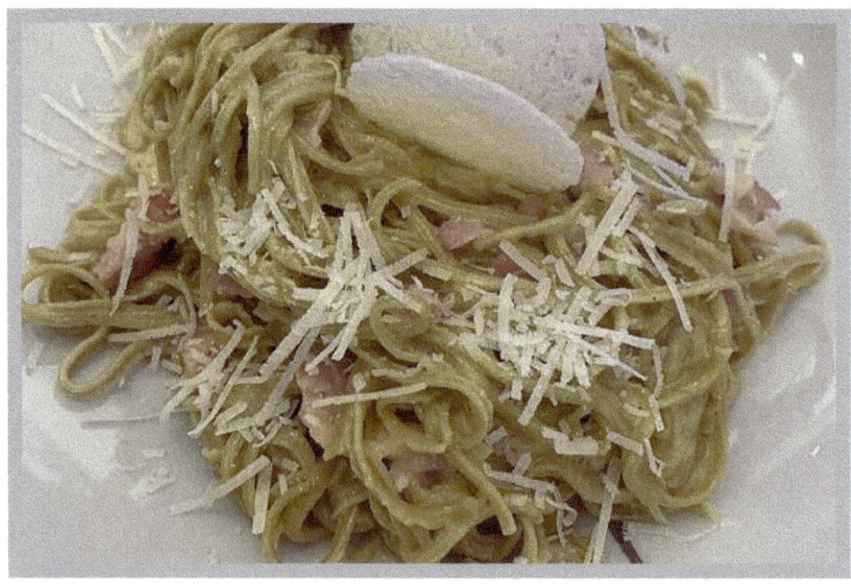

5 MINUTES.
Easy
954 kcal

INGREDIENTS

2 servings

- 150 g spaghetti (soy noodles)
- 200 g cooked ham
- 100 g bacon, cut into strips
- 200 ml of cream
- 4. Egg yolks
- 60 g freshly grated parmesan
- N. B. Oil
- N. B. Salt and pepper
- N. B. Parsley, mild

NUTRITIONAL VALUES per serving
Kcal
954
protein
58.18 g
fat
54.80 gr
carbohydrate
57.57 g

PREPARATION

1. Working time approx. Five minutes

2. Cooking time approx. 15 minutes
3. Total time approx. 20 minutes
4. Cook low-carb pasta according to the directions in the package.

1. In the meantime, dice the bacon strips and the boiled ham and fry them in a very hot pan that has been greased with oil.

1. Beat the egg yolks, about 3/4 of the cream and the grated Parmesan in a bowl and season with pepper and a little salt.

1. Put the still moist spaghetti with the diced bacon / ham in the pan, pour in the rest of the cream and mix with a light spice. Switch off the cooking zone! Now quickly add the egg yolk mixture to the pan, mix everything together and season to taste.

1. Arrange the spaghetti carbonara on plates and serve garnished with parsley leaves.

11
RED LENTIL PASTA

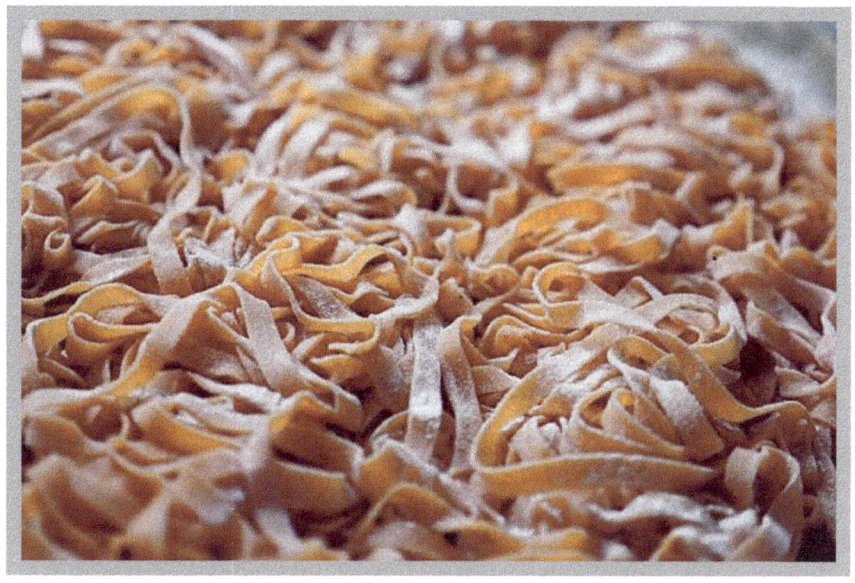

5 minutes.
 Easy

. . .

INGREDIENTS

2 servings

- 250 g lentil flour, red
- Measure 1 egg (s), m
- 1 teaspoon of salt
- 2 teaspoons of olive oil
- 2 pinches of ground nutmeg
- 4 tablespoons of water

PREPARATION

1. Working time approx. Five minutes
2. Rest time approx. 20 minutes
3. Cooking time approx. 3 minutes
4. Total time approx. 28 minutes
5. Mix the dry ingredients well and shape a bowl in the center. Beat the egg with olive oil and a little water. Pour the mixture into the well of the flour mixture and knead by hand. The consistency should be similar to that of the shortcrust pastry. Then let the dough rest for about 20 minutes.

1. After resting the fresh dough, divide it in two and roll it out with a rolling pin until it is the thickness of a matchstick. If the batter is sticky, a little lentil flour can help.

1. Use a pizza pan to cut the rolled dough into thin strips of about 0.5 cm. The width depends on the taste.

1. To cook, add soft crude oil to boiling salted water or let it dry in the oven at approx. 50 °C with the oven door open. 60-90 minutes.

1. The cooking time is about three minutes in the raw state and about six minutes in the dry state; It's important to give it a try if you want it to be al dente.

12

ZUCCHINI NOODLES "GARLIC AND OIL"

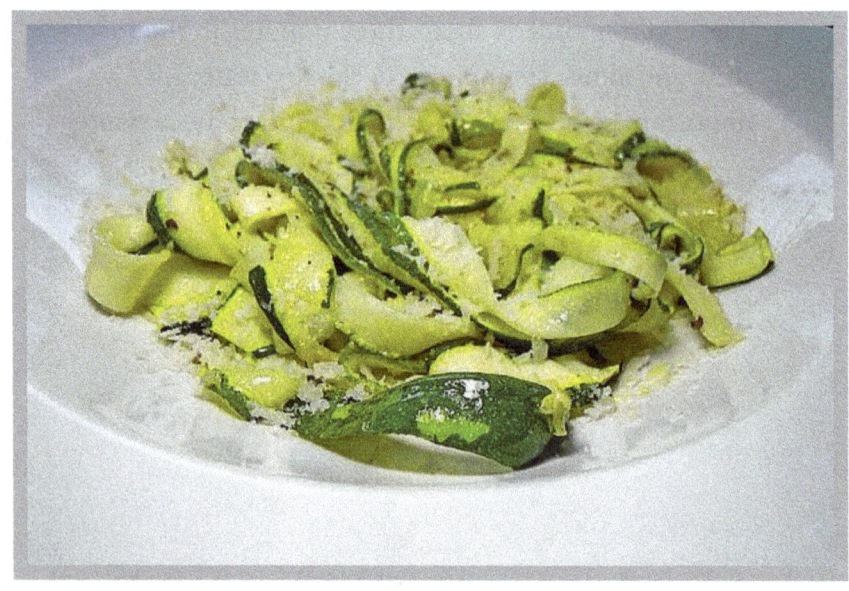

20 MINUTES.
Easy
324 kcal

. . .

INGREDIENTS

2 servings

- Zucchini 3 m tall
- 3 m garlic cloves)
- 3 tablespoons of olive oil
- salt and pepper
- 2 tablespoons of crème fraîche, optional
- 2 tablespoons of Italian herbs (tk), optional
- 2 tablespoons of grated parmesan cheese, optional

Nutritional values per serving

Kcal

324

protein

11.71 g

fat

21.73 g

carbohydrate

19.95 g

PREPARATION

1. Working time approx. 20 minutes
2. Cooking time approx. 10 minutes
3. Total time approx. 30 minutes

4. Cut off the ends of the washed zucchini. Then cut the zucchini lengthways with a julienne cutter into long, thin strips and set aside.
5. In a nonstick pan, heat the olive oil and peel and finely chop the garlic cloves. Fry the garlic in olive oil, just don't let it brown (or it will become bitter!). Reduce the heat to low and throw in the zucchini strips.
6. Cook the zucchini noodles for about 10 minutes, twisting them occasionally so they are firm until they are bitten. Season with salt and pepper.
7. If you like the classic "garlic and oil", you can remove the zucchini noodles from the pan with a fork and place them on a plate.
8. For the variant with a little sauce: add 2 tablespoons of fresh cream, 2 tablespoons of Italian herbs and 2 tablespoons of grated Parmesan, heat briefly and serve.

13
LOW-CARB SPAETZLE

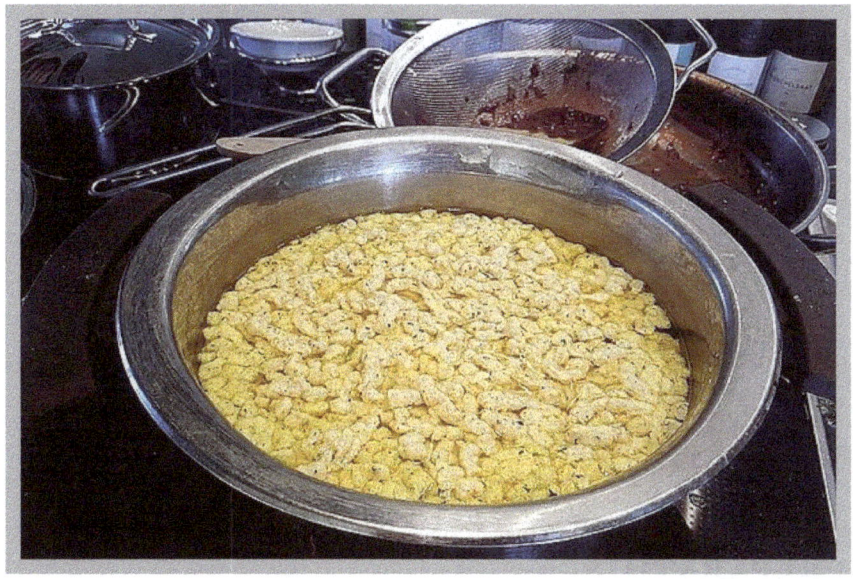

5 MINUTES.
   Easy
   299 kcal

. . .

INGREDIENTS

1 servings

- 100 g of quark
- 20 g of psyllium husk
- 25 g of protein powder, tasteless
- salt and pepper
- Dried parsley
- 25 ml of water
- 1 egg (s)

NUTRITIONAL VALUES per serving

Kcal

299

protein

40.90 g

Fat

11.37 g

carbohydrate

7.59 g

PREPARATION

1. Processing time about 5 minutes
2. Cooking time / cooking approx. 15 minutes
3. Total time about 20 minutes

4. combine every of the ingredients together with a whisk until a smooth batter forms, then soak for 15 minutes.
5. Fill a high-sided saucepan halfway with salted water and bring to a boil.
6. Spread the hard but spreadable dough on the spaetzle grater in hot water. Stir the spaetzle once and remove it from the water with a skimmer.
7. It goes well with a strong sauce, p. Ex. B. A cheese sauce.

14
LOW-CARB DUMPLINGS

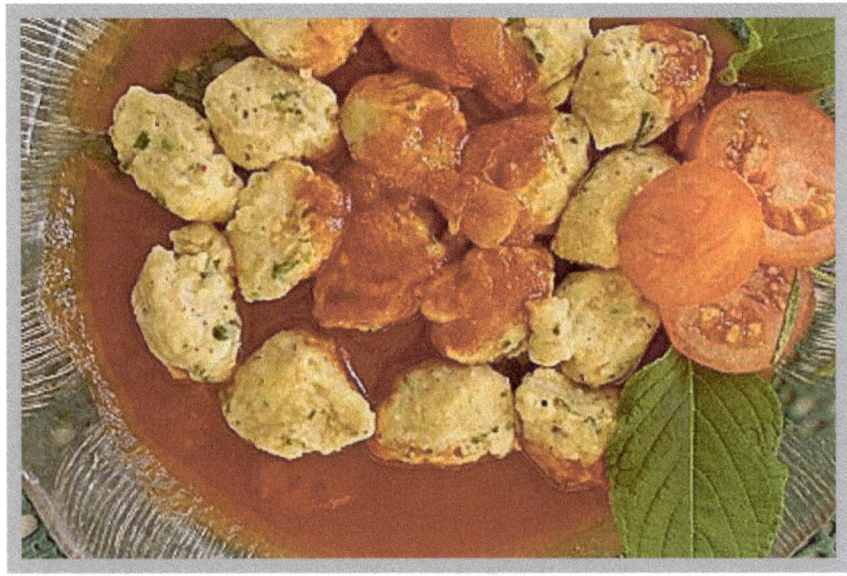

15 MINUTES.
   Easy
   443 kcal

INGREDIENTS

2 servings

- 300 g of cottage cheese
- 1 egg (s)
- 2 egg yolks
- 30 g of wholemeal flour
- 20 g of gluten
- 1 teaspoon of salt
- 1 pinch of pepper
- 1 pinch of nutmeg

Nutritional values per serving
Kcal
443
protein
29.76 g
Fat
28.63 g
carbohydrate
16.85 g

PREPARATION

1. Processing time about 15 minutes
2. Rest time about 30 minutes

3. Cooking / cooking time about 3 minutes
4. Total time about 48 minutes
5. Combine evryof the ingredients in a mixing bowl until a smooth dough forms, then chill for at least 30 minutes.
6. In a large saucepan, bring salted water to a boil, then remove the gnocchi from the batter with two teaspoons and put them in the boiling water. Cook for 3 minutes over medium heat, or until the gnocchi rise to the top.
7. Serve with pasta sauce.

15

HOMEMADE LOW CARB EGG NOODLES WITH TURKEY HAM AND CREAM CHEESE SAUCE

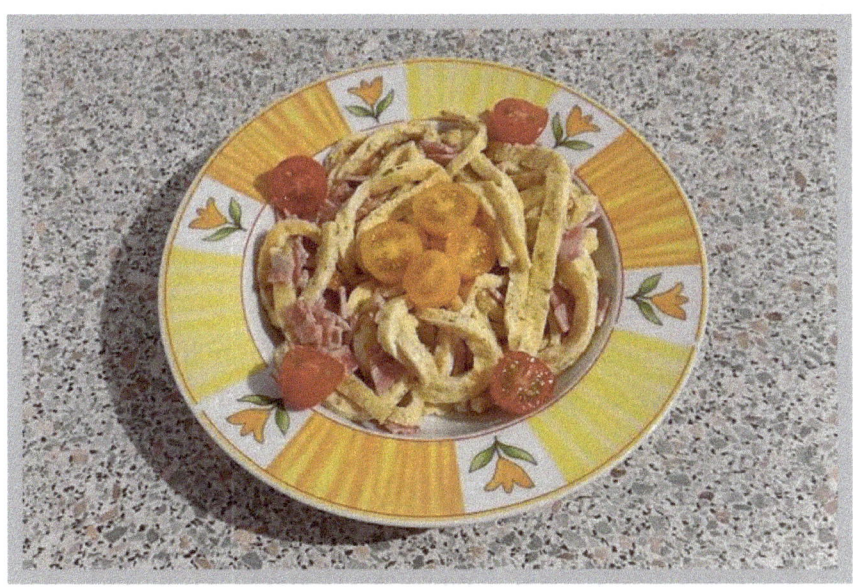

30 MINUTES.

Normal

. . .

INGREDIENTS

1 servings

- g psyllium husks, ground
- 2 eggs)
- 50 g of low-fat cottage cheese
- 1 tablespoon of oregano
- 1 tablespoon of cream cheese
- tablespoons of milk
- 1 tablespoon of oregano
- 4 slices of turkey ham (turkey beer ham)
- 1 tablespoon of sunflower oil

PREPARATION

1. Processing time about 30 minutes
2. Rest time about 10 minutes
3. Cooking / cooking time about 20 minutes
4. Total time about 1 hour
5. For the ribbon noodles, place the psyllium husks, eggs, low-fat quark and oregano in a bowl and mix well.
6. Spread the mixture uniformly over a baking sheet lined with parchment paper in the shape of a rectangle. Pre-heat oven to 160 degrees Celsius and bake for 15 minutes. Allow to cool for 10-15 minutes after removing from the oven.
7. Cut the noodles with a pizza rolling pin.
8. Dice the turkey ham with the beer and set aside.

9. Mix the cream cheese, milk and oregano in a cup.
10. Inside a pan, heat the sunflower oil and fry the noodles. Add the turkey and beer ham and cover with the cream cheese sauce. Simmer for about 5 minutes, stirring occasionally, until the sauce is no longer absorbable by the noodles.

16

LOW CARB GREEN BEANS WITH SHIRATAKI NOODLES

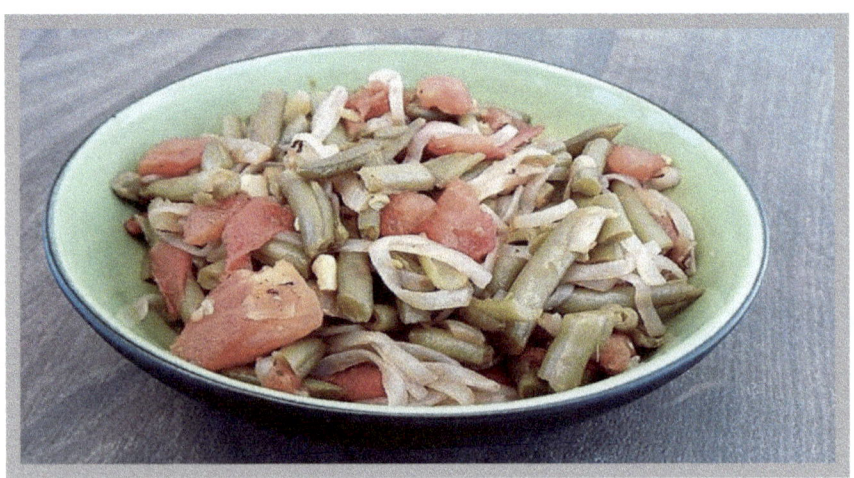

15 MINUTES.
   Simple

INGREDIENTS

4 Servings

- 1 can french beans
- 2 large tomatoes)
- 1 m.-large onion (noun)
- 2 toe / n garlic
- 1 pck. Shirataki noodles
- Oil
- Soup spice (herb soup spice)

PREPARATION

1. Working time approx. 15 minutes
2. Cooking / baking time approx. 15 minutes
3. Total time approx. 30 minutes
4. Dice the onion, wet a pan with oil and preheat on the stove. Fry the onions.
5. In the meantime, drain the green beans and noodle. First add the noodles to the onions and continue frying, then add the green beans. Cut the tomatoes into fine wedges and halve them crosswise again, put them in the pan, sprinkle with herb soup spices, press the garlic through a garlic press and add to the pan. Put the lid on and cook for a few minutes.
6. It tastes best with a roast as a side dish or lightly sprinkled with parmesan as a main course.

⬤17

LOW CARB SPAGHETTI BOLOGNESE WITH SHIRATAKI NOODLES

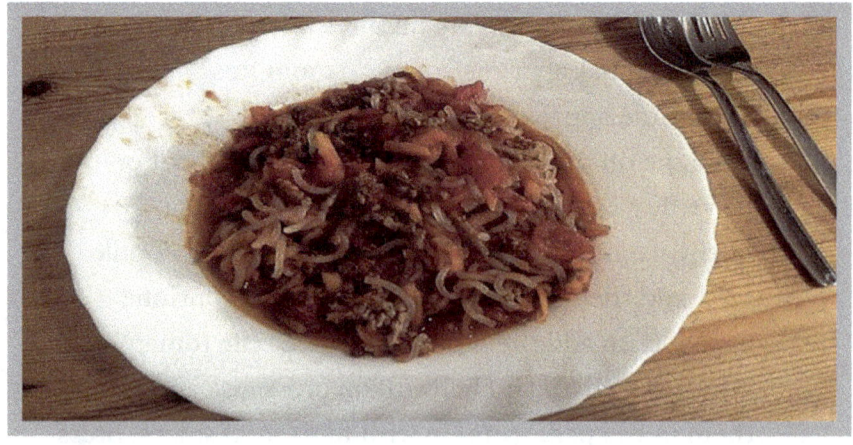

10 MINS.
Normal
150 kcal

INGREDIENTS

1 servings

- 1 small onion
- 50 g carrots
- 1 pack of Shirataki noodles
- 1 can of tomato (s), peeled
- 60 g minced meat (vegetarian minced meat), p. Ex. B. From Quorn
- ½ pack of naturally delicious Knorr! Spaghetti Bolognese (spice base)

PREPARATION

1. Working time approx. 10 minutes
2. Cooking time approx. 30 minutes
3. Total time approx. 40 minutes
4. Chop the onion, grate the carrot and fry both together in 1 teaspoon of olive oil. Add 1 glass of water and cook the vegetables until cooked. Chop 1 can of peeled tomatoes and add. Season to taste with herbs, salt and chilli. Add 1/2 package of base dressing and bring to a boil. Finally add the rinsed shirataki and 60 g Quorn minced beef.

1. The portion is about 150 kcal.

18

LOW CARB LASAGNE WITH PASTA DISHES AND BECHAMEL SAUCE MADE FROM SOY FLOUR

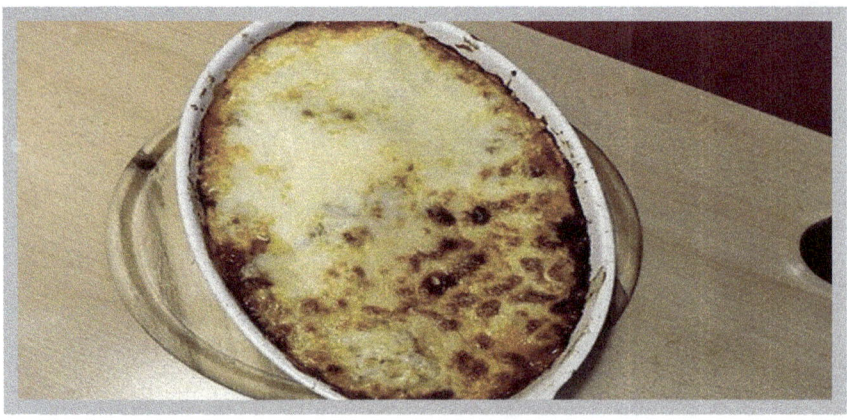

45 MIN.
   normal

INGREDIENTS
   3 servings
   For pasta:

- 200 g soy flour
- Egg (s) 2 m. Large
- 1 pinch of salt
- For the bechamel:
- 25 g soy flour
- 25 g butter
- 300 ml of milk
- salt and pepper
- Some nutmeg

For the Bolognese:

- 400 g of minced meat
- 800 g tomatoes cut into pieces
- salt and pepper
- herbs of Provence
- 1 clove of garlic)
- 1 onion (s), red
- Some oil for frying and for the pan
- Possibly. Grated parmesan cheese

PREPARATION

1. Working time approx. 45 minutes
2. Cooking time approx. 40 minutes
3. Total time approx. 1 hour and 25 minutes
4. Prepare a smooth work surface for the dough. Put the flour on the work surface and make a source. Add a pinch of salt and place the eggs in the center of the

hole.

1. Knead the dough until everything has come together into a uniform dough. The dough must be compact enough. Add a little more flour if necessary.

1. Divide the dough into at least 3 equal portions and roll each portion about 2 mm thick, about the size of the pan. Put aside.

1. For the bechamel, bring the milk to a boil in a saucepan. Melt the butter in another saucepan and add the soy flour. Now slowly pour in the hot milk, stirring constantly, until there are no more lumps.

1. The sauce should have a thick consistency. Season the finished sauce with a little nutmeg, salt and pepper.

1. For the Bolognese, cut the onion into cubes. Chop the garlic or press it into the sauce later.

1. In a saucepan, heat very less oil and fry the onions until they are translucent. After that, attach the minced meat and cook until it is softly pink. Before adding the diced tomatoes, season with garlic, salt, pepper, and Provence herbs to taste.

1. Let the sauce simmer until it is thick and the water no longer separates from the tomatoes.

1. Using oil, grease a pan. Apply a thin layer of Bolognese sauce to the bottom of the pan. To get a light "grill," drizzle a little bechamel sauce over the sauce. The bechamel does not fully cover the Bolognese.
2. Put a pasta dish on top and layer everything in the pan until all of the pasta dishes are gone.

1. Finish with Bolognese and Béchamel. This time we cover the Bolognese completely with the bechamel. Finally, you can sprinkle the grated parmesan on top. Bake the lasagna in a ventilated oven at 200 °C for 15-20 minutes until golden brown.

19

LOW-CARB KELP SPAGHETTI PIZZA WITH TOMATO AND MOZZARELLA

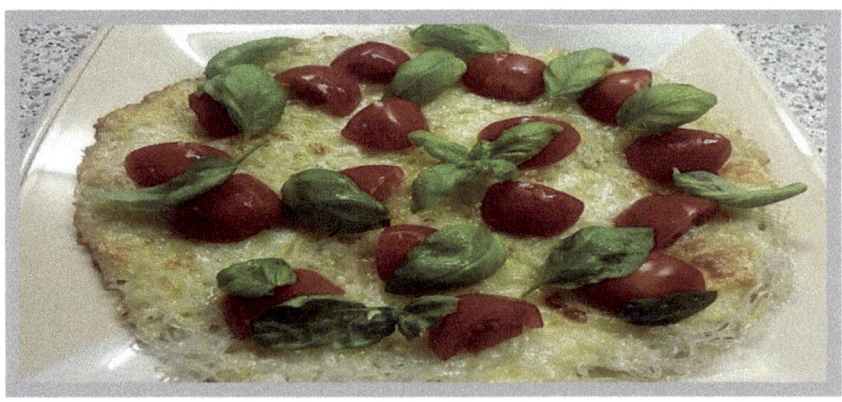

10 MIN.

Normal

INGREDIENTS

1 Servings

KETO PASTA

- 150 g seaweed noodles (kelp noodles)
- 1 m-large egg (s)
- 2 tbsp milk
- 60 g gouda, grated
- 1 ball mozzarella
- Salt and pepper
- Some cocktail tomatoes
- Something basil
- Something butter

PREPARATION

1. Working time approx. 10 minutes
2. Cooking / baking time approx. 15 minutes
3. Total time approx. 25 minutes
4. Preheat the oven to 200 ° c fan-assisted air.

1. Rinse the kelp noodles (half of the package) well with water in a sieve and let them drain.

1. In the meantime, whisk the egg with the milk, salt and pepper and mix in the grated cheese. Cut the cocktail tomatoes into small pieces, drain the mozzarella well and cut into thick slices. Pour off any leaked liquid.

1. Melt the butter in an ovenproof pan (without a plastic handle) on the stove. Put the kelp noodles in the pan and tear them apart with your fingers so that they are evenly distributed. Spread the egg and cheese mixture evenly over the pasta and mix a little carefully, this is a bit tricky. Fry for about 2 - 4 minutes on a medium heat. Don't stir! The bottom should be lightly browned and you should be able to lift it up with a spatula. Now distribute the mozzarella on the seaweed spaghetti.

1. Place the pan in the oven and bake to the desired brown color. This takes about 8 to 12 minutes. You can as well turn on the grill for 2 minutes at the end.

1. Take out the pan, spread the tomatoes and a few leaves of basil on it. Possibly add a little salt. Alternatively, after searing on the stove, the pizza can also be baked on the baking sheet (with baking paper).

1. And don't worry, the noodles neither taste like

seaweed nor are they slimy, you can rather compare them to glass noodles. They don't need to be cooked and are very healthy.

20
ZUCCHINI NOODLES WITH PUMPKIN BULGUR SAUCE

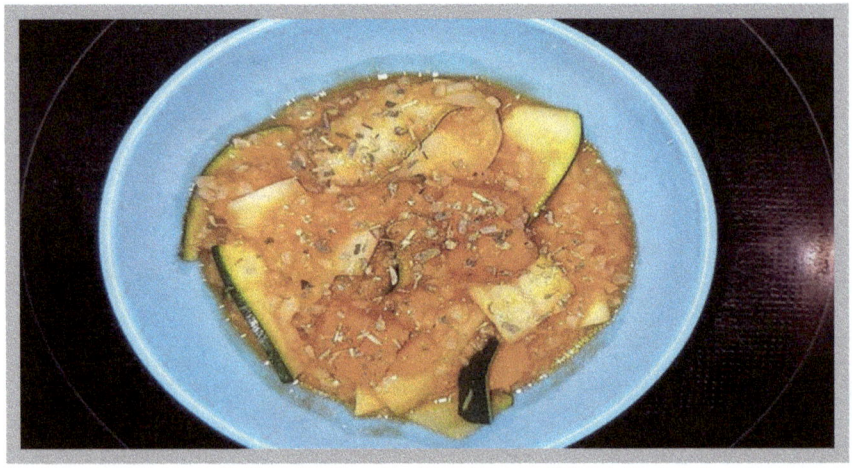

20 MIN.
- Simple

. . .

INGREDIENTS

2 Servings

- 2zucchini
- 250 gbutternut squash (s), pitted
- 75 gbulgur (replace gluten-free or low carb with quinoa)
- 500 mlbroth
- 1 tbsp, heapedtomato paste
- 2 tbspyeast flakes
- onion (noun)
- Salt and pepper
- Herbs, italian

PREPARATION

1. Working time approx. 20 minutes
2. Cooking / baking time approx. 15 minutes
3. Total time approx. 35 minutes
4. If necessary, peel, core and dice the pumpkin. Cut the zucchini into spaghetti with a spiral peeler or into ribbon noodles with a peeler and set aside.

1. Peel and dice the onion and sauté in a little oil until translucent. Add the pumpkin cubes and fry briefly. Simmer with the bulgur and the broth for about 10

minutes. Then add tomato paste, season with salt, pepper, herbs and yeast flakes and finally mix in the zucchini strips.remain o the stove for a few more minutes so that the zucchini is cooked a little.

21
SUMMERY LOW CARB PASTA SALAD

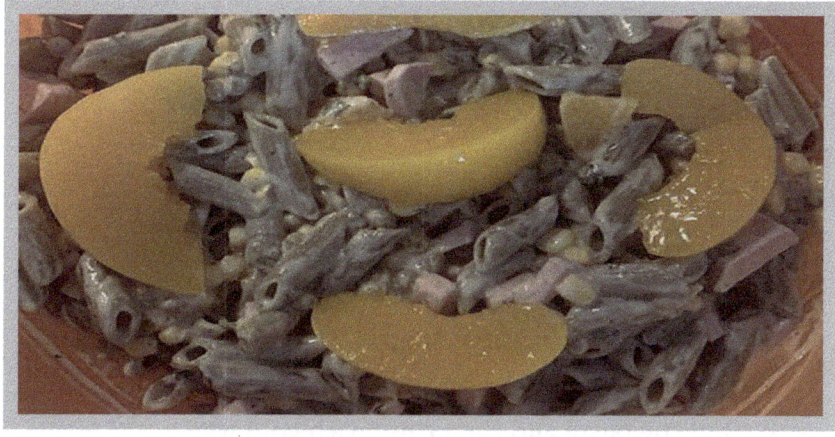

25 MIN.
Simple

INGREDIENTS
8 Servings

- 400 gpenne, made from peas, organic
- 1 cupnatural yogurt, low in fat
- ½ canpeach (s)
- 1 canpeas
- ½ cancorn
- ½ glasssalad mayonnaise (balance)
- 1 splashlemon juice
- Somethingmustard, milder
- 1 bag / nspice mixture (salad topping) italian style
- 250 gpoultry sausage
- ½ fretparsley
- 2 tbsp, heapedcurry powder
- 1 splashvinegar
- Possibly.Apple cider vinegar

PREPARATION

1. Working time approx. 25 minutes
2. Rest time approx. 2 hours
3. Cooking / baking time approx. 10 minutes
4. Total time approx. 2 hours 35 minutes
5. Boil the pasta and then rinse with cold water.
6. Cut the poultry sausage into small pieces.
7. For the dressing, drain the corn, peaches (collect the juice here) and peas and place in a bowl, the salad mayonnaise and yogurt with peach juice from the tin, a splash of lemon juice, some mustard, the lettuce, the chopped parsley and the mix the curry powder. If you

really desire, you can also add a dash of apple cider vinegar.
8. When the pasta has cooled down, add it to the bowl with the dressing and sausage and fold in. Then chill for at least 2 hours.

22

LOW-CARB PASTA SALAD

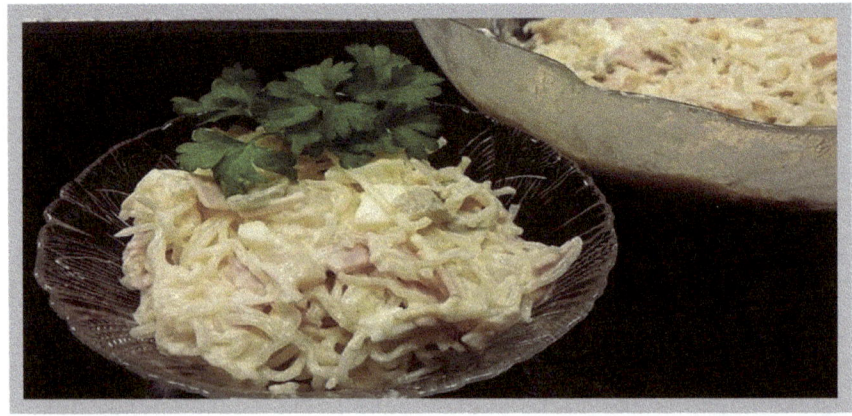

10 MINUTES.
Easy

INGREDIENTS
1 servings

- 1 pack of seaweed spaghetti (seaweed noodles)
- 120 g of cooked ham, cut into thin slices
- 4 m cucumber (jar)
- 3 large, hard-boiled eggs
- 1 glass of small asparagus
- 1 small glass of mayonnaise or salad cream
- salt and pepper
- Possibly. Fresh parsley

PREPARATION

1. Processing time about 10 minutes.
2. Rest time about 10 minutes.
3. Total time about 20 minutes
4. Wash the seaweed noodles well in a colander under running water and let them drain. Cut the pasta into small pieces, no need to cook, put them in a bowl. Cut the ham, peeled eggs and cucumber into cubes, drain the asparagus and cut into small pieces. Add everything to the pasta in the bowl. Add salt and pepper, and then stir in the mayonnaise. If required, chop the parsley into small pieces and combine with the other ingredients.

1. Pasta salad can be eaten after 10 minutes.

1. But it can also be kept in the refrigerator for at least 3 days so that it can be prepared well. The pasta is very crunchy. Ideal for parties or work. Great solution to a low carb diet to get back to eating pasta salad.

23

TANDOORI CHICKEN WITH SHIRATAKI NOODLES (KONJAK NOODLES)

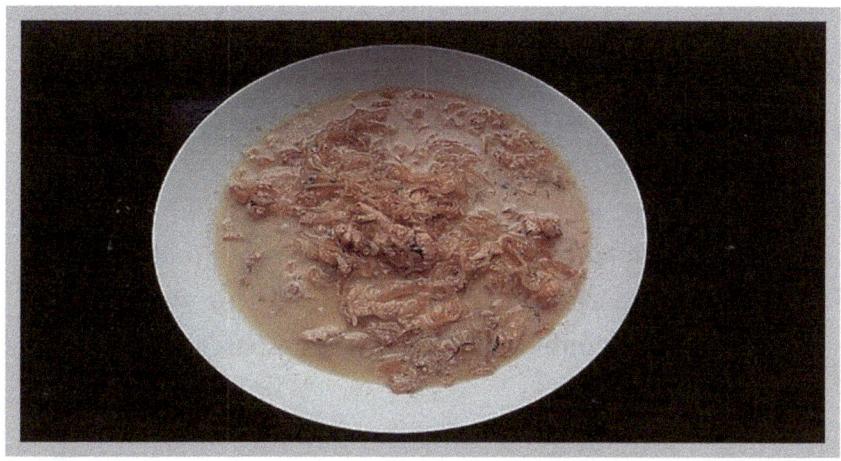

15 MINUTES.
Easy

INGREDIENTS
1 servings

- 1 chicken breast fillet (s)
- N. B. water
- 1 onion
- 1 teaspoon of beef broth, immediately
- 2 teaspoons of tandoori masala
- 100 g of noodles (Shirataki or Konjak)
- 50 g of cheese (Harzer with noble rot)
- 1 slice (s) of fresh ginger
- 2 leaves of wild garlic
- 200 g of skimmed milk (0.1% fat)
- salt
- kilos

PREPARATION

1. Processing time about 15 minutes
2. Total time about 15 minutes
3. scrape and quarter the onion and cut into thin strips. Simmer in a saucepan covered with a little water, the broth and tandoori masala until transparent.

1. Wash the shirataki in a colander (untangle and chop if necessary) and add them to the onions in the pan. If necessary, add more water so that nothing burns. Let it simmer for 5 minutes.

1. In the meantime, rinse the chicken breast under cold water, pat it dry and cut it into strips. Also add to the pan and cook, stirring occasionally.

1. Finely chop the ginger, cut the wild garlic into thin strips and chop the resinous cheese into small pieces. Put everything in the pan and mix well until the resinous cheese has melted (be careful, it burns quickly!).

1. Now turn off the heat and add the yogurt, stir briefly and let it heat up, but not too much, otherwise the yogurt will flocculate. add taste with salt and chilli and serve.

1. The recipe is suitable for all phases of the Dukan diet. For a vegetarian meal, I recommend adding quartered cherry tomatoes.

24

HAZELNUT SAUCE WITH BEETS AND RED LENTIL NOODLES

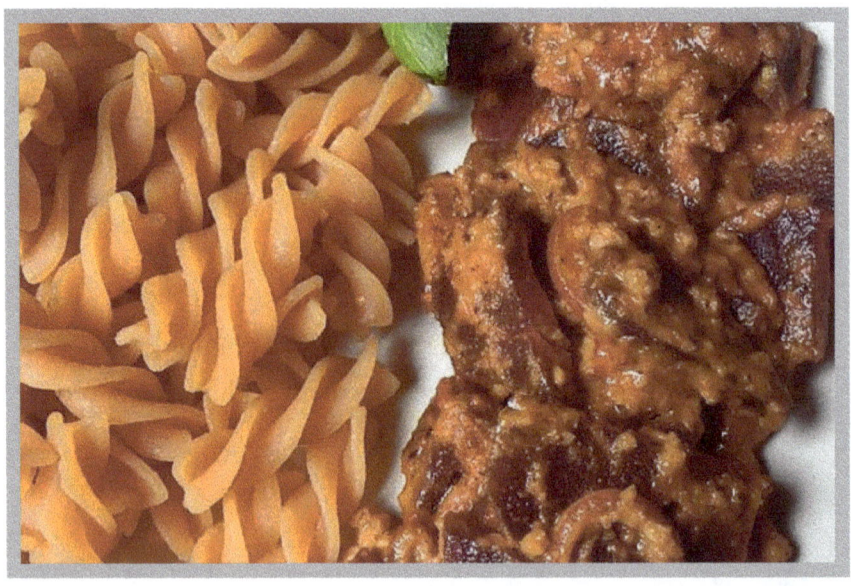

10 MINUTES.

Easy

. . .

INGREDIENTS

1 servings

- 150 g of lentil noodles (red lentil noodles, for example from dm)
- 1 heaping tablespoon of butter
- 1 onion
- 1 clove of garlic, optional
- 3 cooked beet bulbs
- 50 g of chopped hazelnuts
- 100 ml of water
- A little turmeric
- A little paprika powder, nobly sweet.
- Something salty
- A little stevia or some other sweetener
- Possibly. cream
- Parsley for garnish

PREPARATION

1. Processing time about 10 minutes.
2. Cooking time / cooking approx. 15 minutes
3. Total time about 25 minutes
4. Put the water for the pasta in a saucepan.
5. Leave the butter in a pan. Meanwhile, cut the onion into rings or finely chop it to taste and sauté it in a pan until translucent. If you want you can also add a clove of garlic cut into small pieces.

1. Put the pasta in the salted cooking water and cook over medium heat according to the manufacturer's instructions.

1. Cut the cooked beets into fork-sized pieces.

1. Add the chopped hazelnuts to the onion rings in the pan and continue cooking over medium heat. With about 100 ml of water. Add turmeric, paprika powder, salt and sweetness as needed and season to taste. A little sweetness enhances the flavor and binds any bitter substances that may be present. If you really want, you can add a drop of cream or something similar.
2. Add the beets to the sauce in the pan and simmer to heat them. Reduce everything a little if there is too much liquid.

1. Drain the pasta and serve with the sauce. Garnish with some chopped parsley or something similar.

1. If you don't like beets, you can just omit or substitute them.

1. My test diner, who doesn't like low carbs, wants the dish to cook this way again!

25

RADISH AND WALNUT SAUCE WITH ZUCCHINI NOODLES

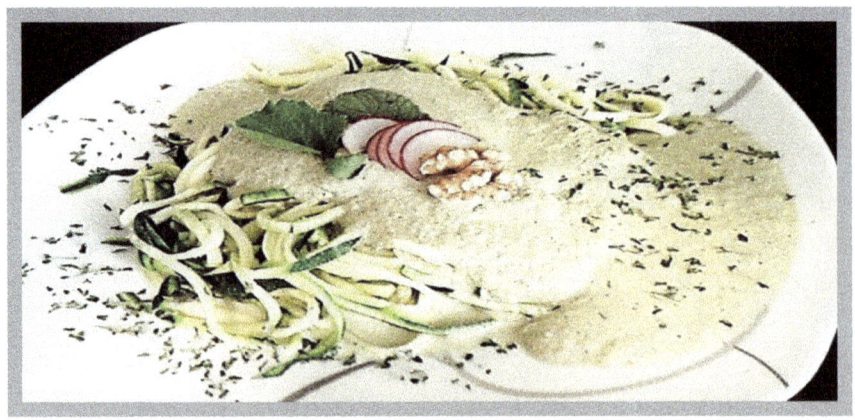

20 MINUTES.
Easy
266 kcal

INGREDIENTS
4 servings

- 1 bunch of radishes and vegetables, approx. 320 g
- 3 zucchini
- 1 onion
- 80 g walnuts
- 100 g soy cream (cooking based on soy cream)
- 2 tablespoons of lemon juice
- 250 g of water
- 1 teaspoon thyme
- 1 teaspoon paprika powder, flavorful like a rose
- 1 teaspoon of salt
- ½ teaspoon pepper
- 20 g of oil
- N. B. water
- N. B. Sal

NUTRITIONAL VALUES per serving
Kcal
266
protein
9.67 g
fat
21.11 g
carbohydrate
9.12 g

PREPARATION

1. Working time approx. 20 minutes

2. Cooking time approx. 20 minutes
3. Total time approx. 40 minutes
4. First wash the radishes and their leaves. scrape the onion, cut in half and put in a mixing bowl, chop for 5 sec. / Speed 5, then press with a spatula. Add 20 g of oil and simmer for 2:30 min / varoma / speed 1.

1. Then add radishes with leaves and 80 g walnuts to the onions and chop 5 sec / speed 5, put everything back in and add 250 g water. This actually based on the size of the radish bunch. Otherwise, start with less water and water a little later. The mash should be almost covered with water. Let it boil for 10 minutes / set 1/100 ° C.

1. In the meantime, make the zucchini noodles, cut 3-5 zucchini into "tagliatelle" depending on size and hunger. Works best with a peeler or julienne cutter. Now just pour boiling water over the pasta and let it steep for five minutes.

1. When the time is up, mix the sauce gradually, 30 sec / level 6-8-10. Add 100 g of cream, 1 teaspoon of salt and 1/2 teaspoon of pepper and then mix again 20 sec

/ speed 10. If sauce is still too thick, put a little more water or cream.

1. Drain the pasta through a sieve and finally add the thyme, paprika powder and 2 tablespoons of lemon juice to the sauce. Mix again for 10 seconds / speed 3 and season to taste, if necessary.

1. Now it is enough to arrange the pasta on a plate and cover with the sauce and, if necessary, garnish with a little parsley, walnuts or radishes.

TIP: The sauce can be very spicy as I don't season the pasta.

I cooked this amount for two and then poured the rest of the sauce over a green salad. The sauce certainly goes well with normal or gluten-free pasta.

26
CREAMY CUCUMBER AND PEPPER TAGLIATELLE

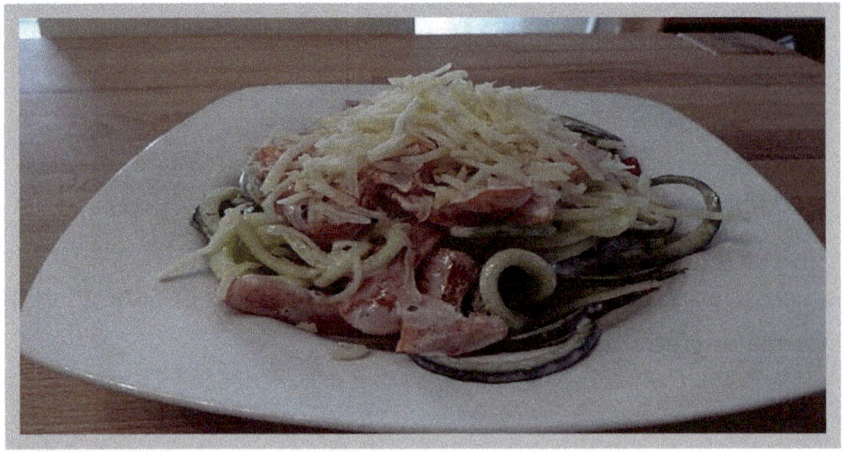

10 MINS.
Easy
609 kcal

INGREDIENTS

2 servings

- 300 g cream cheese
- salt and pepper
- 1 bell pepper
- 1 cucumber
- 100 g emmental

Nutritional values per serving
Kcal
609
protein
28.73 g
fat
51.35 g
carbohydrate
8.22 g

PREPARATION

1. Working time approx. 10 minutes
2. Cooking time approx. Five minutes
3. Total time approx. 15 minutes
4. Put the cream cheese, salt and pepper in a large pan and let it melt over medium heat. Cut the bell pepper into thin, short strips and add to the sauce.
5. Use a spiral cutter to shape the cucumber into

spaghetti. Once the sauce is creamy, add the cucumber noodles to the pan and mix.
6. Once the cucumber is hot, take it out of the pan and spread it on the plates. Grate the cheese and sprinkle with the cucumber and pepper noodles.

27

ZUCCHINI NOODLES WITH CRABS AND VEGETABLES

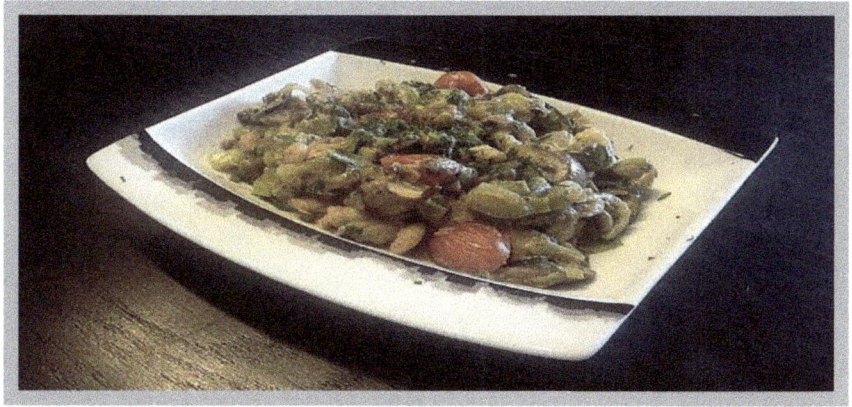

15 MINUTES.
Normal
286 kcal

INGREDIENTS
3 servings

- 2 m of zucchini
- 2 leeks
- 2 small onions
- 2 cloves of garlic
- 250 g of mushrooms
- 250 g of cherry tomatoes
- 80 g of Kat ham
- 100 g of cream cheese
- 300 ml of vegetable broth
- 200 g prawns (sea prawns)
- salt and pepper
- Herbs

Nutritional values per serving
Kcal
286
protein
29.57 g
Fat
12.49 g
carbohydrate
12.87 g

PREPARATION

1. Processing time about 15 minutes
2. Cooking time / cooking approx. 15 minutes
3. Total time about 30 minutes

4. Pass the courgettes through the spiral cutter or cut them into small pieces with the potato peeler and fry them in olive oil. Pour in the vegetable broth, cook for 5 minutes and then set aside.
5. Fry the onions and garlic in olive oil, add the mushrooms, leek and ham and sauté briefly. Then add the tomatoes, shrimp and zucchini and simmer for 5 minutes. Finally add the cream cheese and let it melt. Season the vegetable mixture with herbs, salt and pepper.

1. Food is enough for 3 normal diners or 2 good ones.

1. It is suitable not only for low carbohydrate products but also for low calorie products. If you are not low in carbohydrates and want to cut down on fat, you can opt for lean ham and light cream cheese.

28

CHICKEN WITH ZUCCHINI AND CARROTS

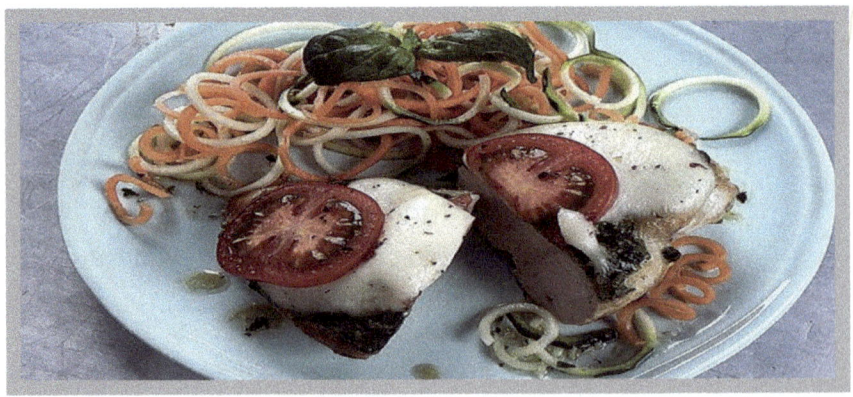

30 MINUTES.
Easy

INGREDIENTS
4 servings

- 800 g of chicken breast
- 2 tablespoons of rapeseed oil
- 2 mozzarella
- 2 large tomatoes)
- Pesto, green
- 3 courgettes
- 3 carrots
- 1 tablespoon of butter
- nutmeg
- Garlic powder

PREPARATION

1. Processing time about 30 minutes.
2. Cooking time / cooking approx. 45 minutes.
3. Total time about 1 hour and 15 minutes
4. Wash the chicken breast, pat dry, season with salt and pepper and fry in 1 tablespoon of rapeseed oil. Put the chicken breast in a saucepan, spread it with pesto and cook for 40 minutes at 200 ° C in the upper and lower parts of the oven.

1. Wash and slice the tomatoes. Also cut the mozzarella into slices. 10 minutes before the chicken breast is cooked, place the tomato and mozzarella slices on the chicken breast and cook at the same time.

1. Wash the courgettes and cut the ends, peel the carrots and remove the ends as well. Transform both into spaghetti with vegetables with the help of a spiral cutter.

1. Fry the carrot spirals in butter with nutmeg. Fry the courgette spirals with salt, pepper and garlic in 1 tablespoon of rapeseed oil to keep them firm until bitten. Mix the zucchini and carrot noodles, remove the chicken breast from the oven, place on the vegetable spaghetti and serve.

ZUCCHINI NOODLES WITH SHRIMP AND TOMATO SAUCE

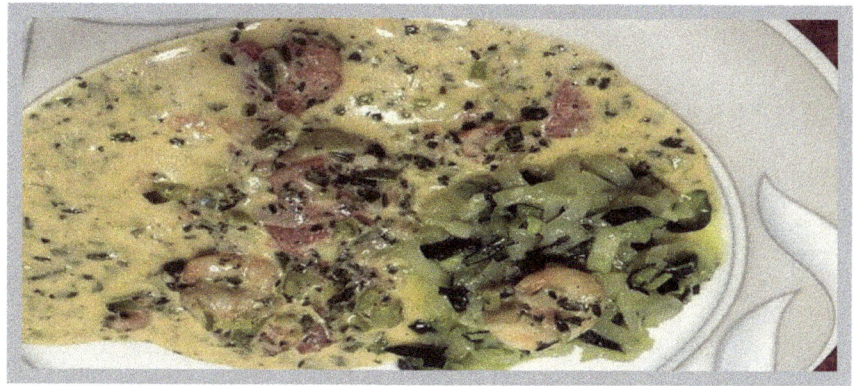

30 MINUTES.
Easy

INGREDIENTS
1 servings

- 120 g of prawns)
- 1 courgette
- 1 large tomato)
- 1 clove of garlic)
- 1 small spring onion)
- basil
- parsley
- Garlic cloves
- salt and pepper
- chili powder
- A little cream
- A little oil
- water

PREPARATION

1. Processing time about 30 minutes.
2. Cooking / cooking time about 20 minutes
3. Total time about 50 minutes
4. Preparation:
5. scrape the garlic and grate it finely with a grater / alternatively chop it finely. Cut the tomatoes, chives and herbs into pieces of your choice and set aside.
6. Since the zucchini here are to be used as a pasta substitute, they are peeled into thin strips with a potato peeler. Then continue peeling and set the zucchini strips aside.

SAUCE:

1. try Heat a little oil in a non-stick pan and fry the prawns and garlic. Now lower the heat and add the tomatoes and chives to the pan and let it simmer for a few minutes.
2. For a nice creamy sauce, add a splash of cream and, if necessary, a little water. As a last step, I seasoned my sauce with salt, pepper and chilli and added the fresh herbs. Now let it rest over low heat.

"TAGLIATELLE":

1. you Boil the water in a saucepan or kettle and then put it in a bowl with the zucchini strips. Come out good. After about 3 minutes, they should be soft and can be poured.

1. Pour the sauce over the "noodles" and serve.

ZUCCHINI NOODLES WITH PRAWNS AND TOMATO SAUCE

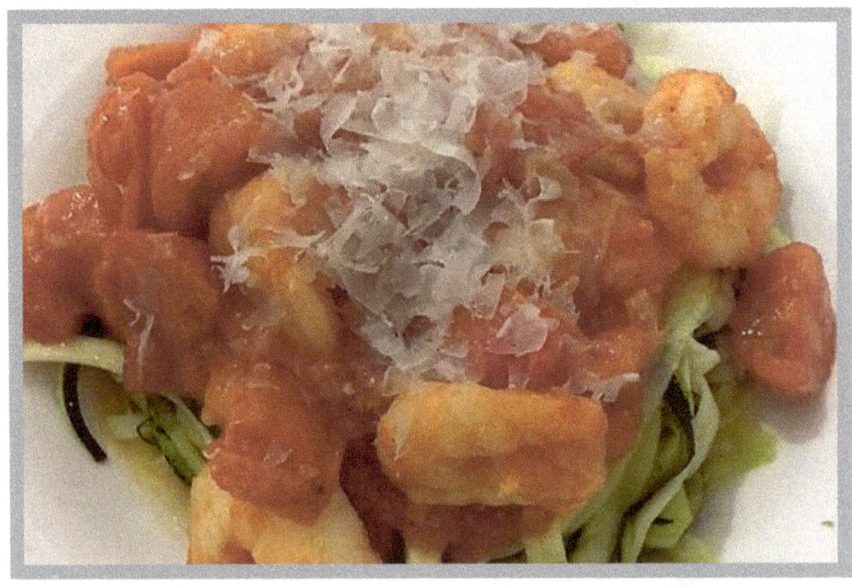

20 MINUTES.

normal

. . .

INGREDIENTS

- servings
- small zucchini
- 18 prawns
- tomatoes)
- 1 onion
- 1 can of diced tomatoes
- Frying oil

PREPARATION

1. Working time approx. 20 minutes
2. Cooking time approx. 15 minutes
3. Total time approx. 35 minutes
4. Wash the zucchini as it will be used with the skin. Use the peeler to cut the zucchini into strips until you reach the grains. The stripes look like green ribbon spaghetti.

1. Then fry the prawns in the oil. You can also use garlic or another oil to do this. Just before cooking, place the prawns on a plate and put the previously chopped tomatoes, chopped onions, and the tin with the chopped tomatoes in the same pan. After 2 minutes over medium heat, return the prawns to the sauce.

Let the sauce simmer for about 5 minutes while you pour the zucchini noodles with boiling salted water. Let it steep for approx. 5 minutes with the lid closed. So that it can be served.

www.ingramcontent.com/pod-product-compliance
Lightning Source LLC
Chambersburg PA
CBHW071117030426
42336CB00013BA/2128